Birth ■ *Naître* ■ Die Geburt

Photographs of Magnum Photos • *Photographies de Magnum Photos* • **Fotografien von Magnum Photos**

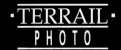
·TERRAIL·
PHOTO

■ Editor: Jean-Claude Dubost
Desk Editor: Caroline Broué in liaison with Magnum Photos' team
Cover design: Gérard Lo Monaco and Laurence Moinot
Graphic design: Véronique Rossi
Iconographic and artistic coordination at Magnum Photos:
Marie-Christine Biebuyck, Agnès Sire, assisted by Philippe Devernay
English translation: Ann Sautier-Greening
Photoengraving: Litho Service T. Zamboni, Verona

© FINEST SA / ÉDITIONS PIERRE TERRAIL, Paris 1998
The Art Book Subsidiary of BAYARD PRESSE SA
© Magnum Photos, Paris 1998
ISBN 2-87939-167-9
English edition: © 1998
Publication number: 200
Printed in Italy

■ *Direction éditoriale : Jean-Claude Dubost*
Suivi éditorial : Caroline Broué en liaison avec l'équipe de Magnum Photos
Conception et réalisation de couverture : Gérard Lo Monaco et Laurence Moinot
Conception et réalisation graphique : Véronique Rossi
Direction iconographique et artistique à Magnum Photos :
Marie-Christine Biebuyck, Agnès Sire, assistées de Philippe Devernay
Traduction anglaise : Ann Sautier-Greening
Traduction allemande : Inge Hanneforth
Photogravure : Litho Service T. Zamboni, Vérone

© FINEST SA / ÉDITIONS PIERRE TERRAIL, Paris 1998
La filiale Livres d'art de BAYARD PRESSE SA
© Magnum Photos, Paris 1998
ISBN 2-87939-165-2
N° d'éditeur : 200
Dépôt légal : mars 1998
Imprimé en Italie

■ Verlegerische Leitung: Jean-Claude Dubost
Verantwortlich für die Ausgabe: Caroline Broué
in Zusammenarbeit mit dem Magnum Photos Team
Umschlaggestaltung: Gérard Lo Monaco und Laurence Moinot
Buchgestaltung: Véronique Rossi
Bildredaktion und grafische Gestaltung für Magnum Photos:
Marie-Christine Biebuyck, Agnès Sire; Assistent: Philippe Devernay
Deutsche Übersetzung: Inge Hanneforth
Farblithos: Litho Service T. Zamboni, Verona

© FINEST SA / ÉDITIONS PIERRE TERRAIL, Paris 1998
Der Bereich Kunstbücher von BAYARD PRESSE SA
© Magnum Photos, Paris 1998
ISBN 2-87939-166-0
Deutsche Ausgabe: © 1998
Verlegernummer: 200
Printed in Italy

"I walked around all day, my mind occupied, seeking on the streets photographs to be taken directly from life as if in flagrante delicto. I wanted above all to seize in a single image the essence of any scene that cropped up. [...] Photography is the only means of expression which freezes one specific instant", wrote Henri Cartier-Bresson, one of the founding members of the Magnum Photos Agency.

During their assignments to the four corners of the earth, the photographers of this prestigious agency have all wanted to record a certain reality directly seized "from life" and to show the world as they saw and felt it. Their photographs bear witness to the experience of men, to places, times and events which their cameras have managed to capture. The personal imprint they leave on them proves, in the words of John Steinbeck, that "the camera need not be a cold mechanical device. Like the pen, it is as good as the man who uses it. It can be the extension of mind and heart...".

The ambition of the series to which this album belongs is to recall the finest of these "decisive moments", where the eye of the photographer encounters the diversity of the world. Whether it is read like a report or looked at like a film, each album is above all a thematic, historic and aesthetic odyssey bringing together the best pictures from the Magnum photographers.

"Je marchais toute la journée, l'esprit tendu, cherchant dans les rues à prendre sur le vif des photos comme des flagrants délits. J'avais surtout le désir de saisir dans une seule image l'essentiel d'une scène qui surgissait. [...] De tous les moyens d'expression, la photo est le seul qui fixe un instant précis », écrivait Henri Cartier-Bresson, l'un des fondateurs de l'agence Magnum Photos.

Les photographes de cette prestigieuse agence ont tous voulu, au cours de leurs reportages à travers le monde, rendre compte d'une certaine réalité « sur le vif » et montrer le monde tel qu'ils le voyaient et le ressentaient. Leurs photos témoignent de l'expérience d'hommes, de lieux, d'époques et d'événements que leur appareil a su capter. L'empreinte personnelle qu'ils laissent prouve, selon les mots de John Steinbeck, que « l'appareil-photo n'est pas nécessairement une froide mécanique. Comme la plume pour l'écrivain, tout dépend de qui la manie. Il peut être un prolongement de l'esprit et du cœur... »

Restituer les plus beaux de ces « instants décisifs » au fil desquels l'œil du photographe rencontre la diversité du monde, telle est l'ambition de la collection dans laquelle s'inscrit ce livre. À lire comme un récit ou à regarder comme un film, il est avant tout une promenade thématique, historique et esthétique qui rassemble les meilleurs clichés des photographes de Magnum Photos.

"Den ganzen Tag lief ich angespannt herum, denn ich wollte in den Straßen wie auf frischer Tat ertappte, lebensnahe Fotos machen. Vor allem hatte ich den Wunsch, in einem einzigen Bild das Wesentliche eines Geschehnisses festzuhalten [...] Von allen Ausdrucksmitteln ist die Fotografie das einzige, das einen bestimmten Augenblick fixiert", schrieb Henri Cartier-Bresson, einer der Gründer der Fotoagentur Agence Magnum Photos.

Den Fotografen dieser renommierten Agentur liegt viel daran, auf ihren Reportagen in aller Welt von einer gewissen „lebensnahen" Realität Zeugnis abzulegen und die Welt so zu zeigen, wie sie sie sahen und empfanden. Die Fotos sind von ihrem Apparat eingefangene Erfahrungen mit Menschen, Orten, Zeiten und Ereignissen. Der persönliche Eindruck, die sie hinterlassen, beweist, um mit Steinbeck zu sprechen, daß „der Fotoapparat keine kalte Mechanik sein muß. Wie bei der Feder des Schriftstellers hängt alles davon ab, wer sie hält. Und manchmal ist es sogar eine Verlängerung von Geist und Gefühl ..." Die schönsten dieser „entscheidenen Augenblicke" zu zeigen, bei denen das Auge des Fotografen der Vielfältigkeit der Welt begegnet, ist die Absicht dieser Buchreihe. Wie ein Bericht zu lesen oder wie ein Film zu betrachten, ist sie vor allem ein thematischer, historischer und ästhetischer Spaziergang, auf dem die besten Bilder der Fotografen von Magnum Photos zu sehen sind.

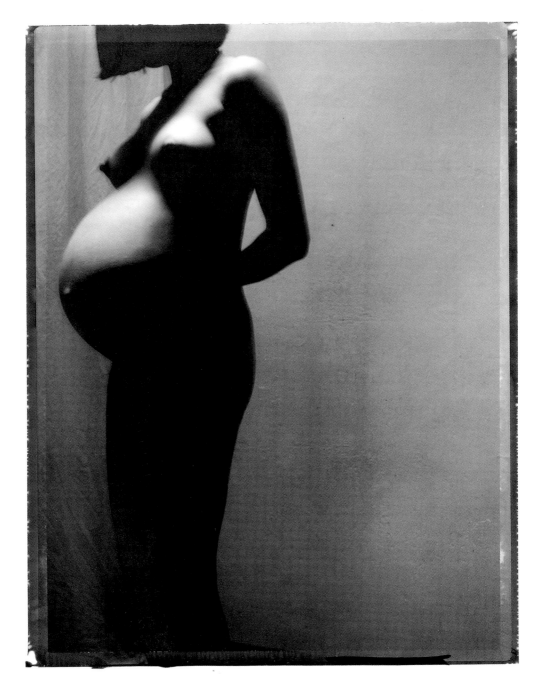

Josef Koudelka, *France,* Frankreich, 1986. **5**

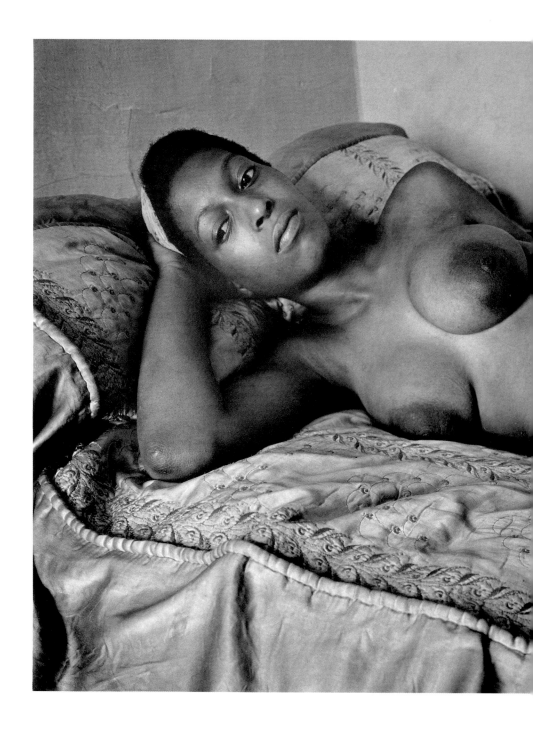

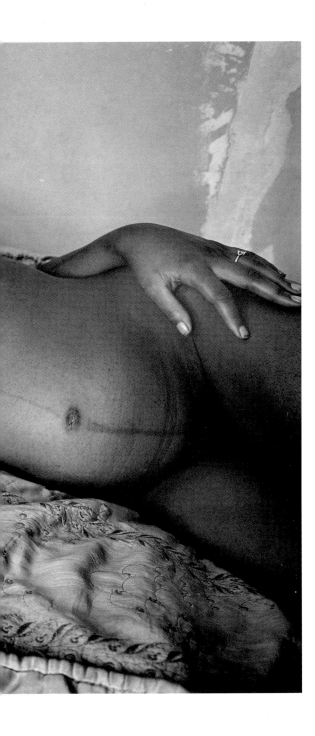

Bruce Davidson, USA, *États-Unis,* 1966-1968. **7**

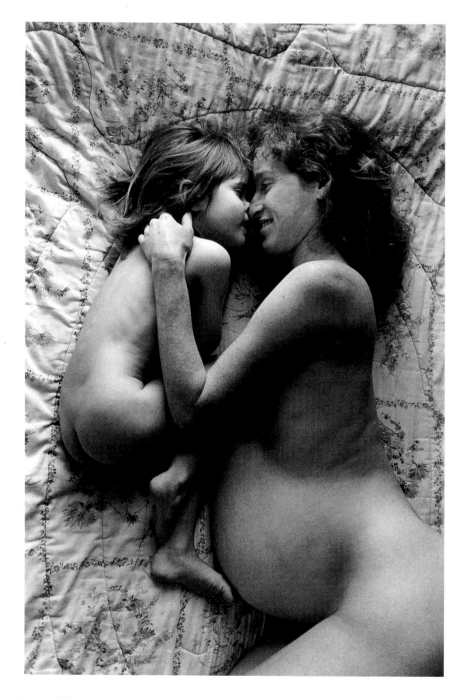

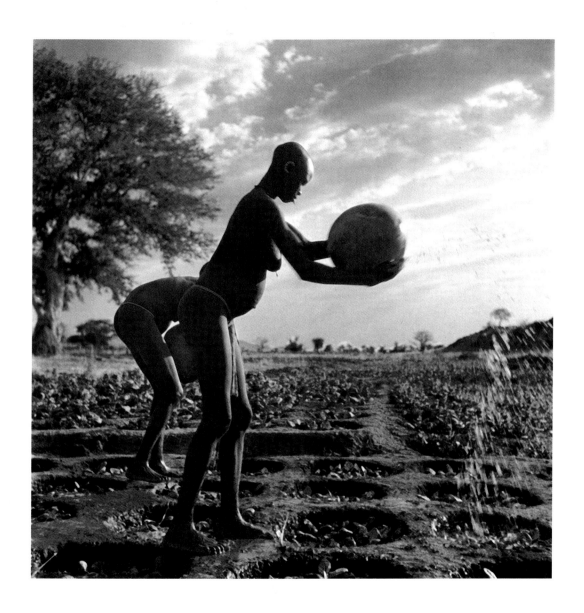

George Rodger, Southern Sudan, *Sud-Soudan,* Südsudan, 1949. | **9**

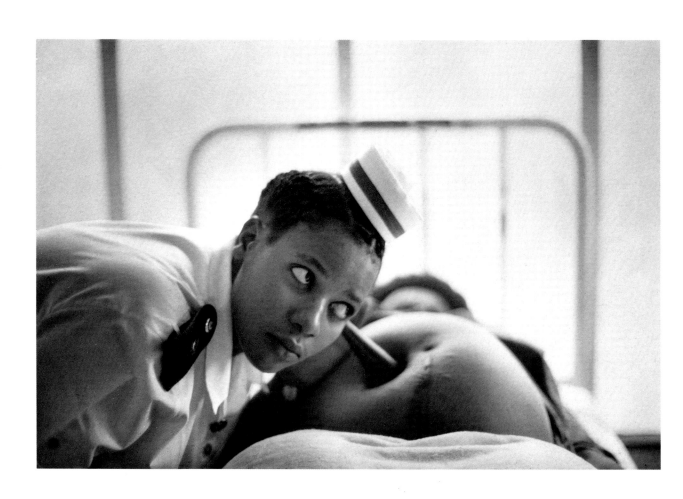

| Eve Arnold, South Africa, *Afrique du Sud,* Südafrika, 1973.

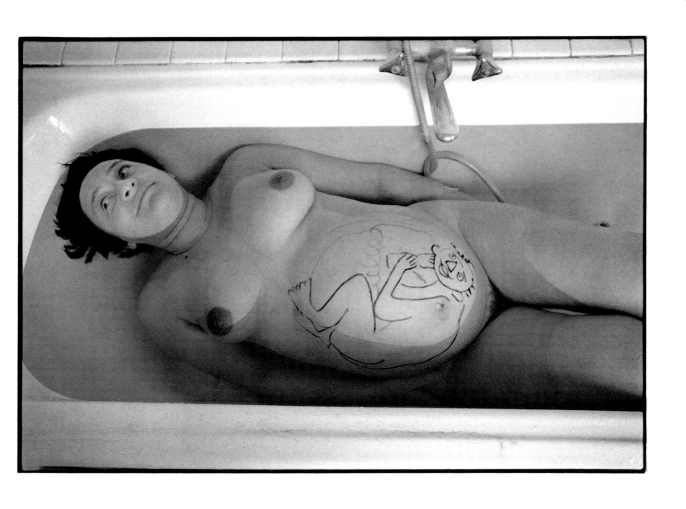

Patrick Zachmann, *France,* Frankreich, 1986. **11**

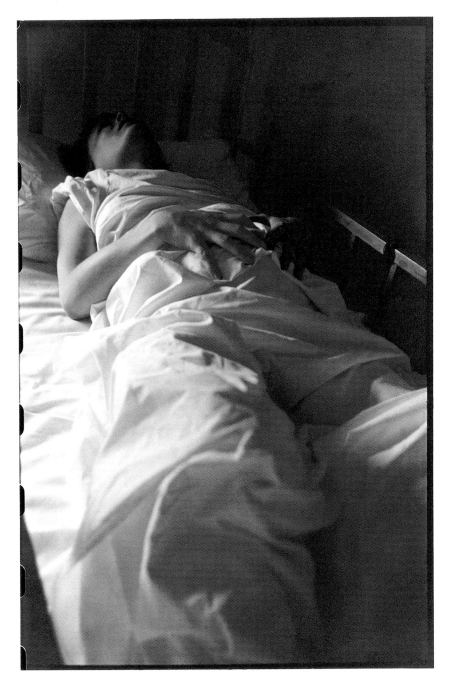

Elliott Erwitt, USA, *États-Unis,* 1972.

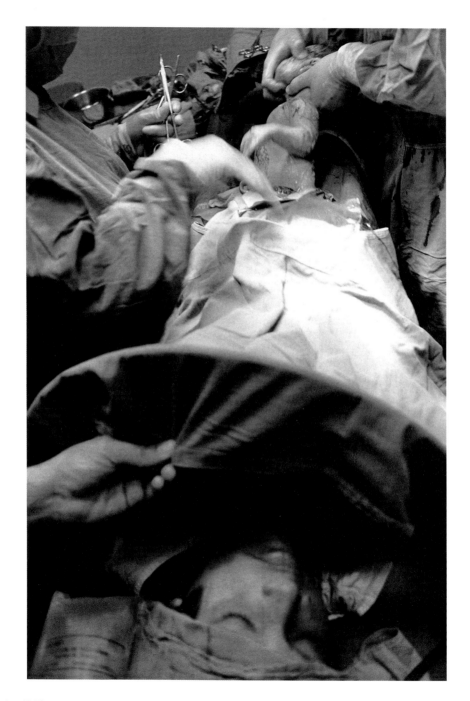

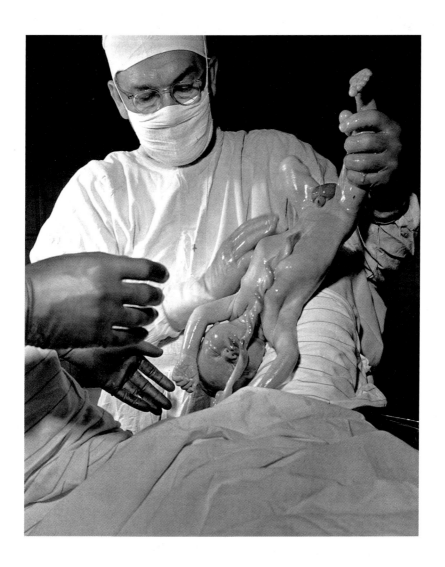

Wayne Miller, USA, *États-Unis,* 1946. **15**

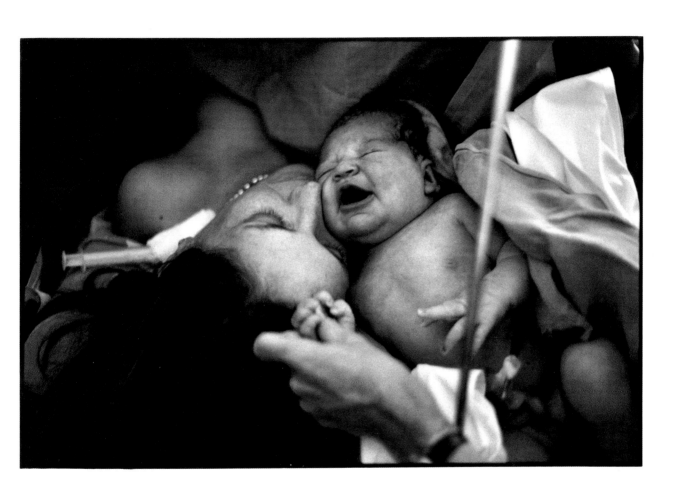

Josef Koudelka, *France,* Frankreich, 1986. | **17**

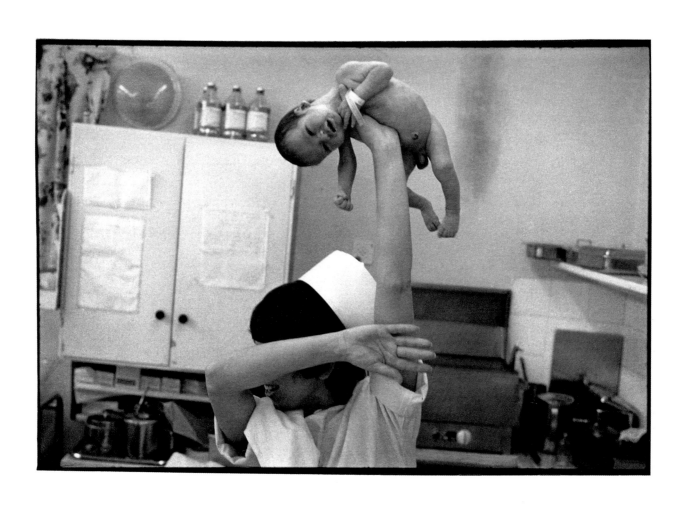

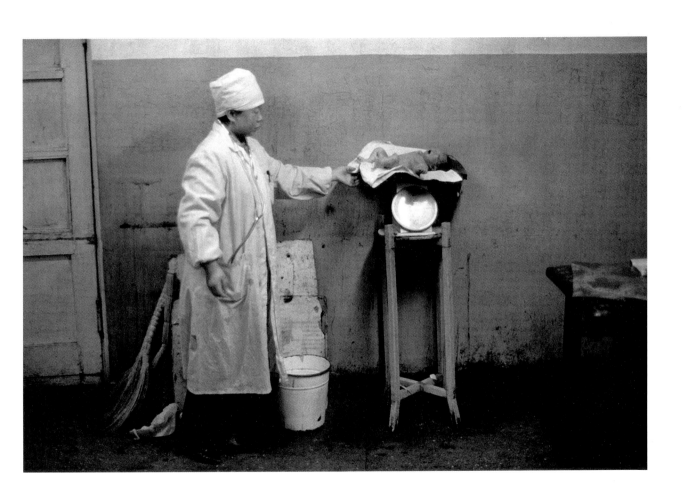

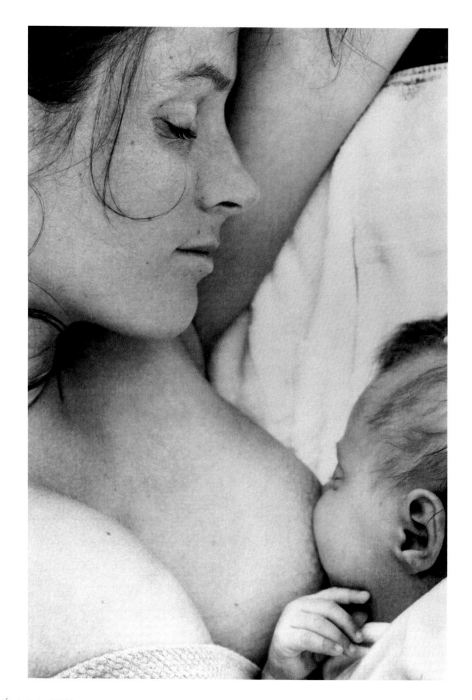

| Elliott Erwitt, USA, *États-Unis*, 1977.

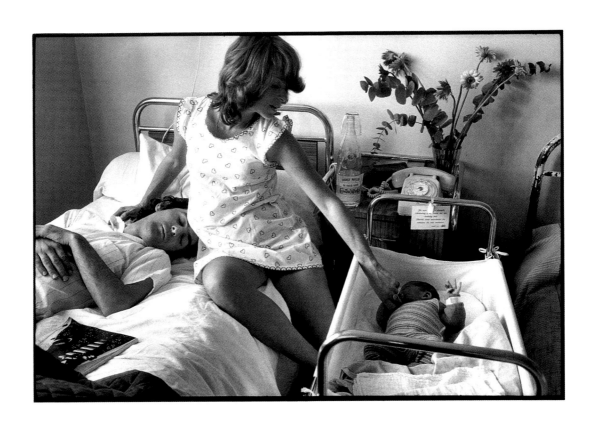

Guy Le Querrec, *France,* Frankreich, 1972. |

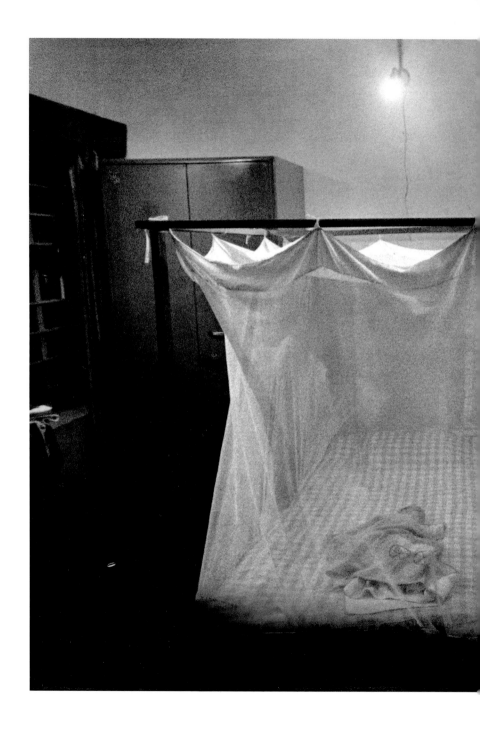

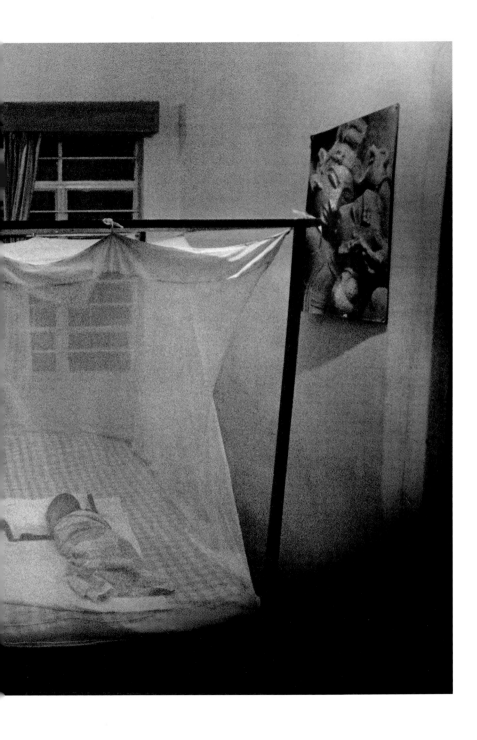

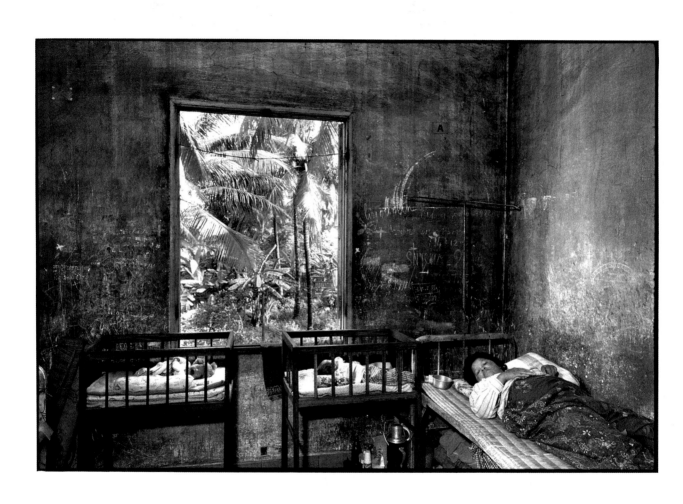

| Patrick Zachmann, Cambodia, *Cambodge,* Kambodscha, 1991.

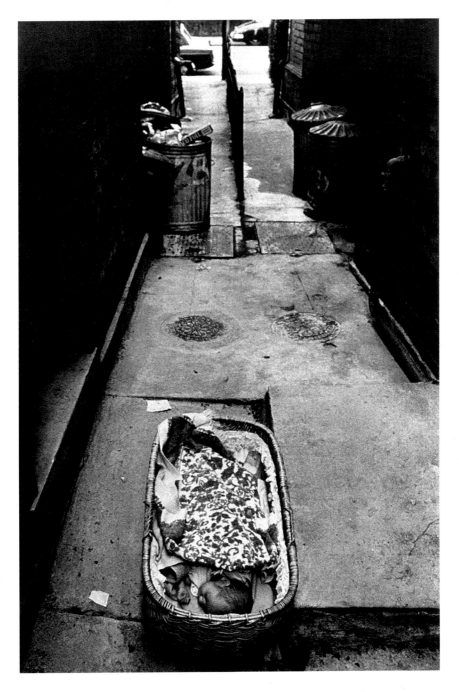

Josef Koudelka, Wales, *Pays de Galles,* 1969.

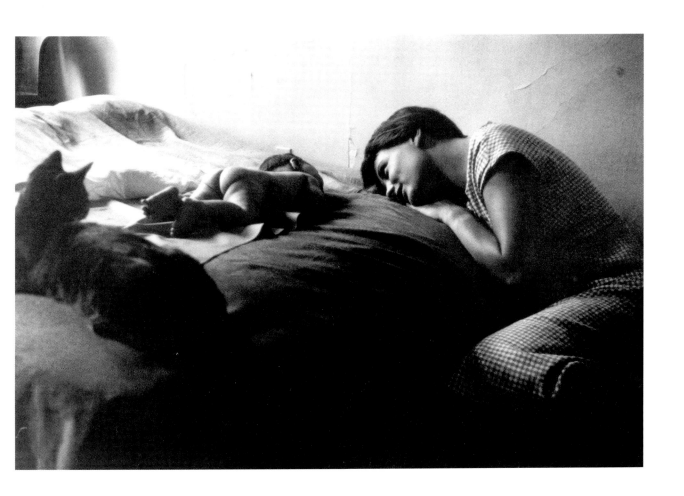

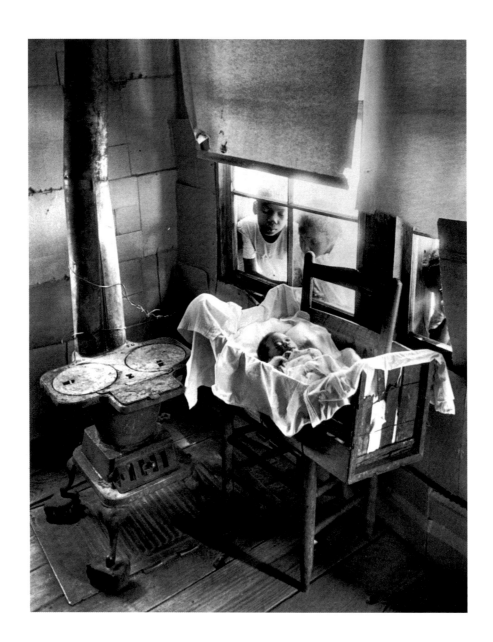

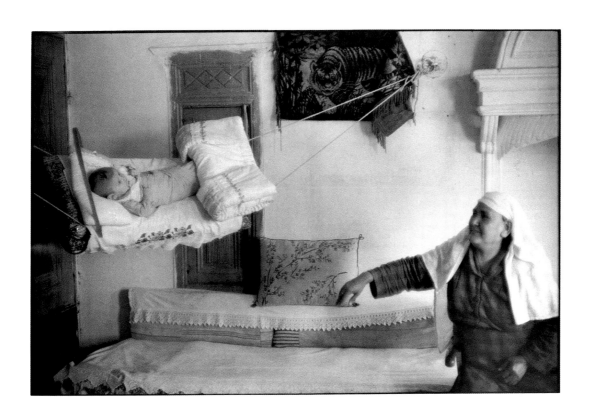

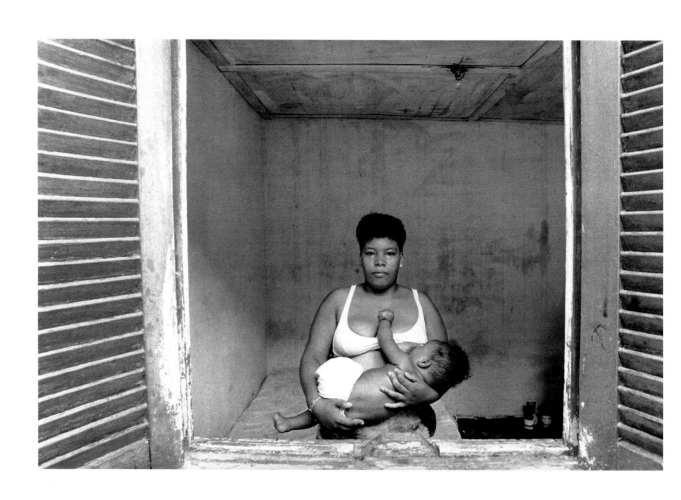

30 | Alex Majoli, Brazil, *Brésil,* Brasilien, 1996.

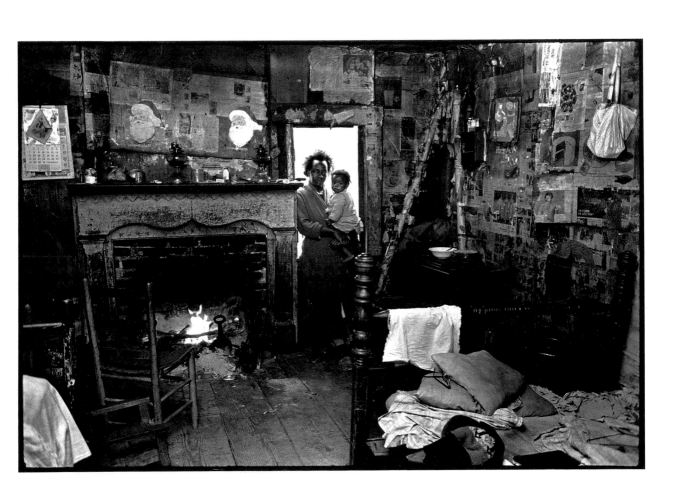

Bruce Davidson, USA, *États-Unis,* 1965. | **31**

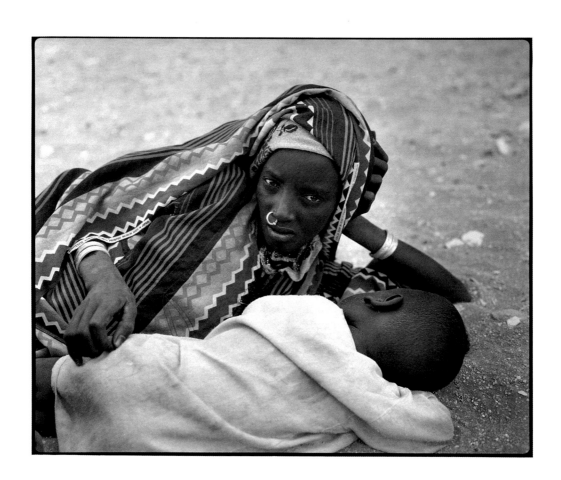

| Raymond Depardon, *Niger,* 1989.

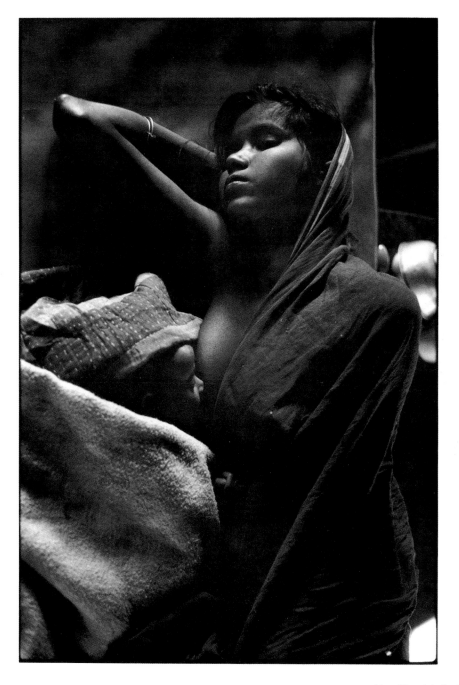

Marc Riboud, India, *Inde,* Indien, 1971. | **33**

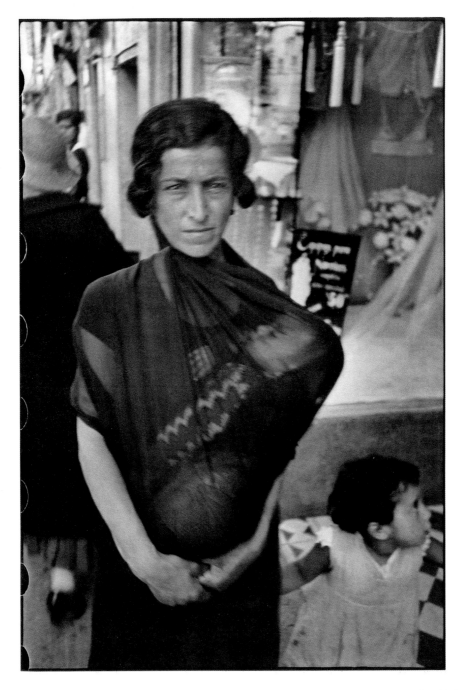

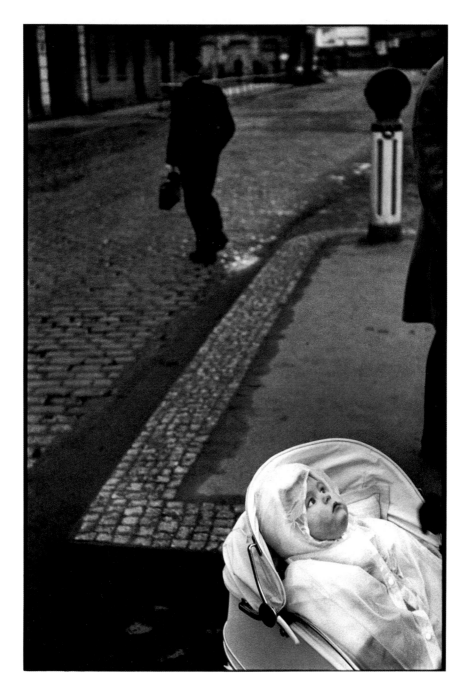

| René Burri, Federal Republic of Germany, *RFA*, Bundesrepublik Deutschland, 1960.

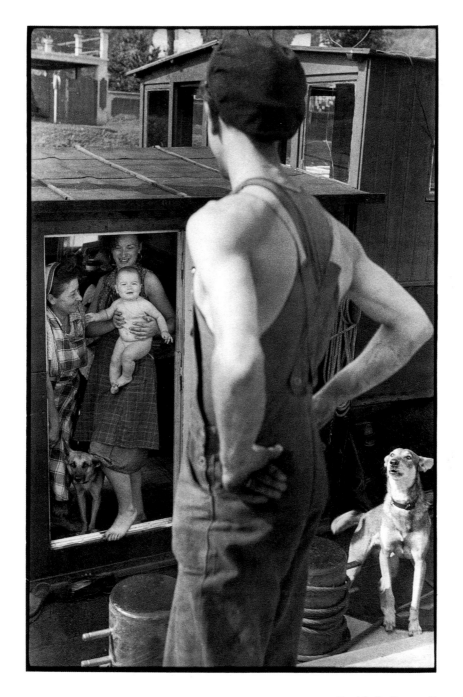

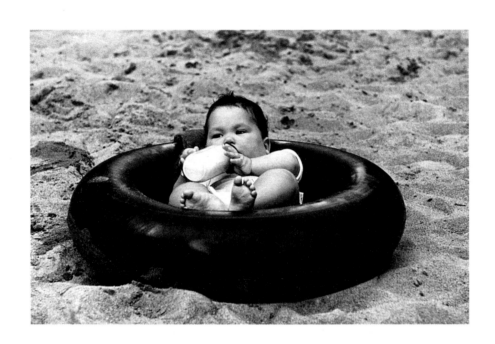

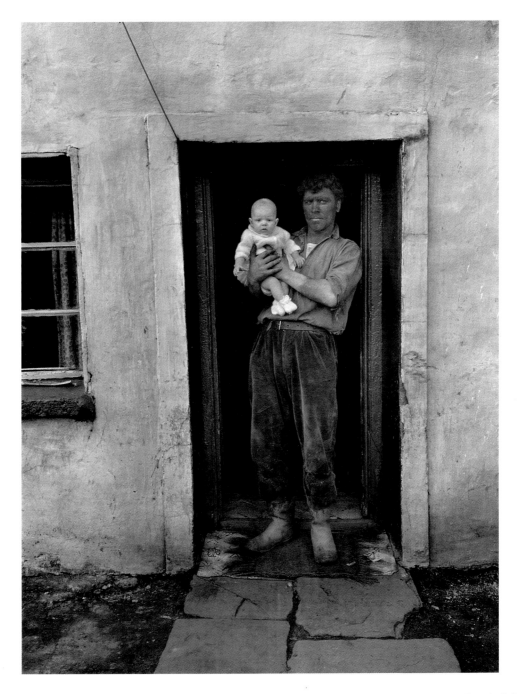

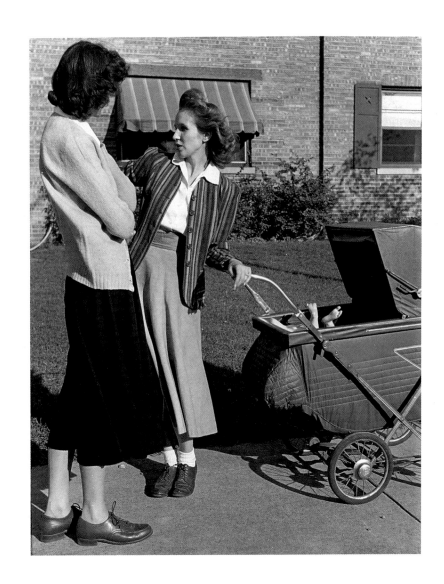

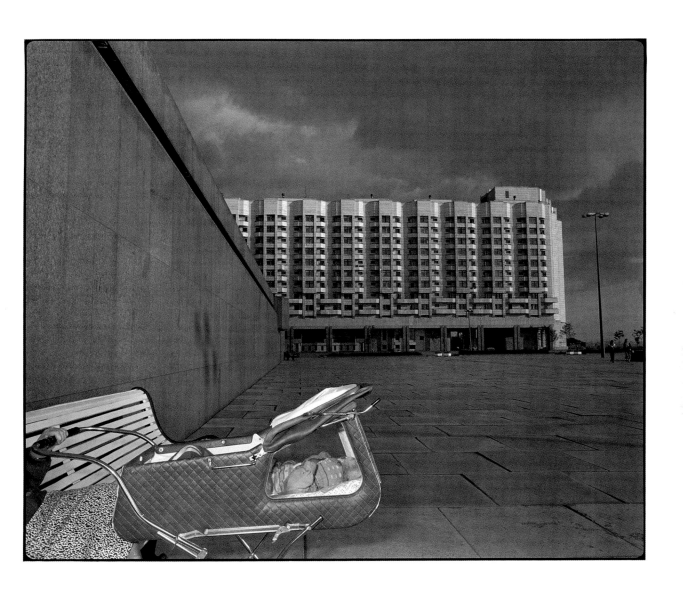

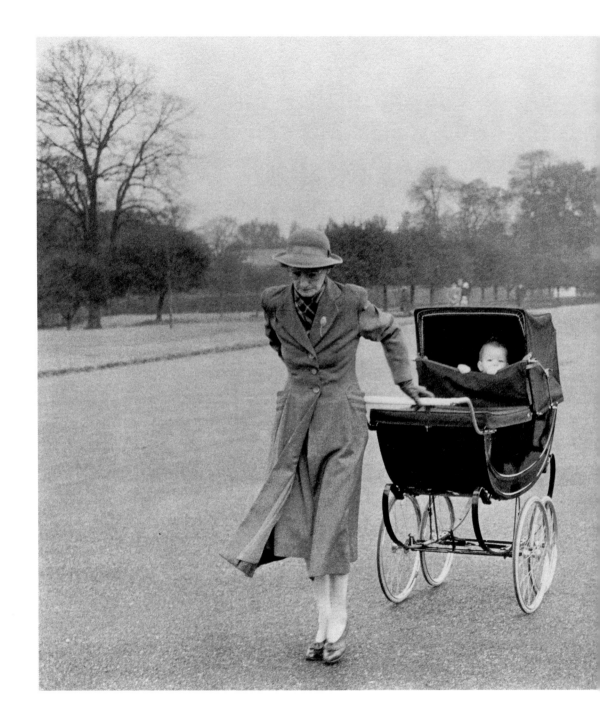

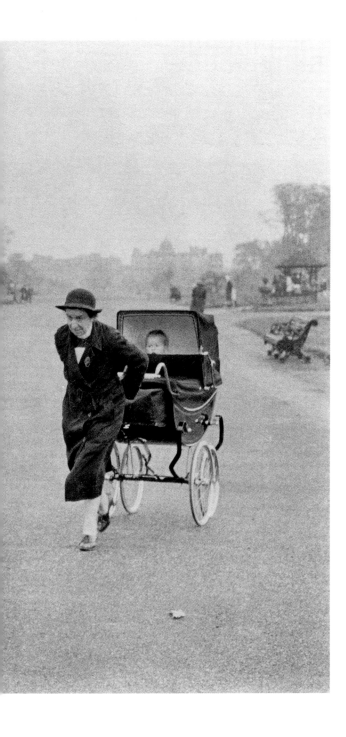

Bruce Davidson, Scotland, *Écosse,* Schottland, 1960.

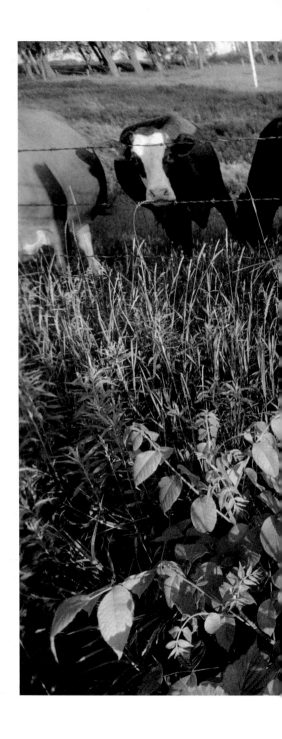

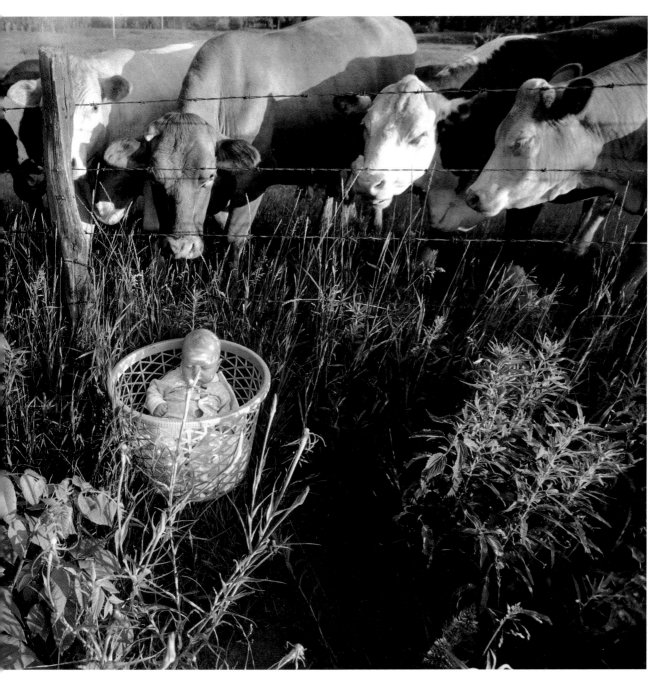

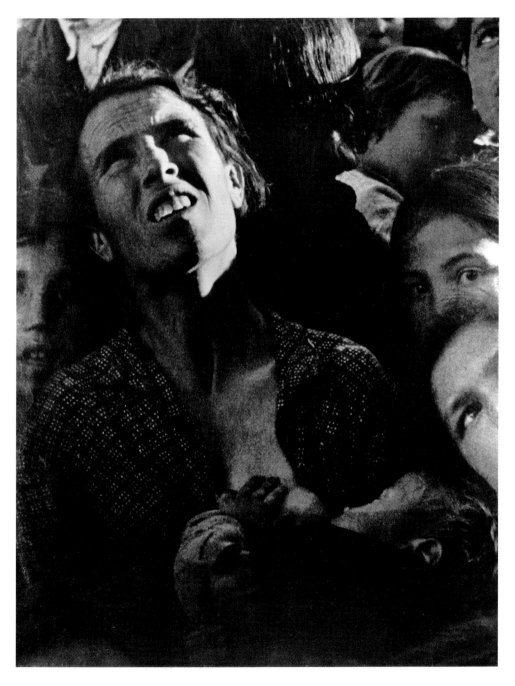

David Seymour, Spain, *Espagne,* Spanien, 1936. **47**

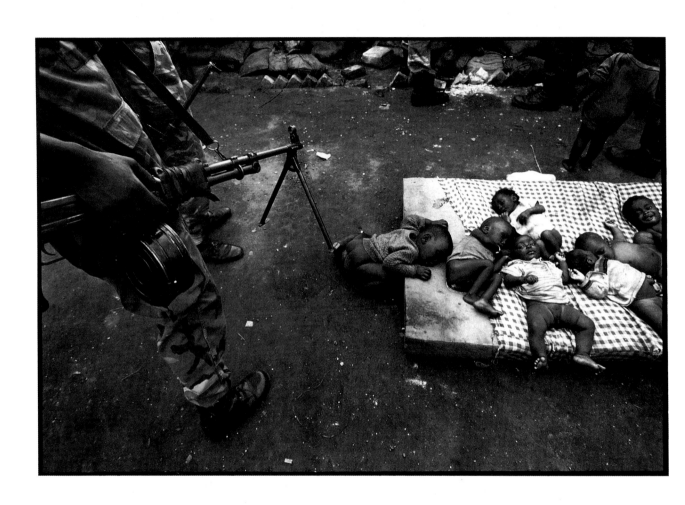

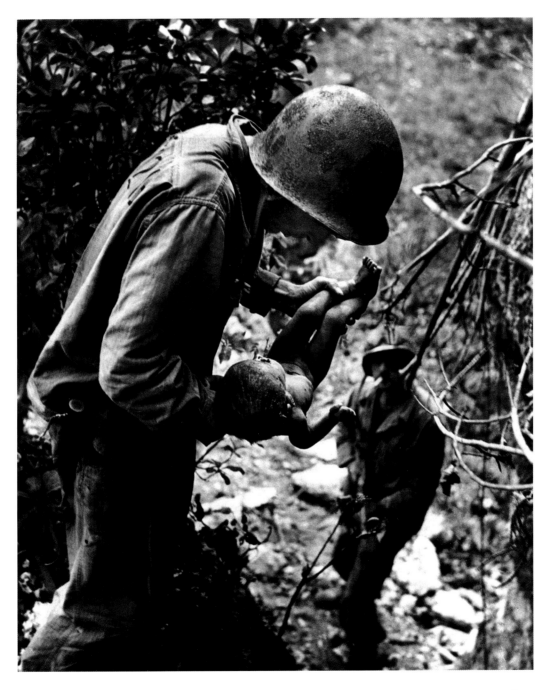

W. Eugene Smith, USA, *États-Unis,* 1944. **49**

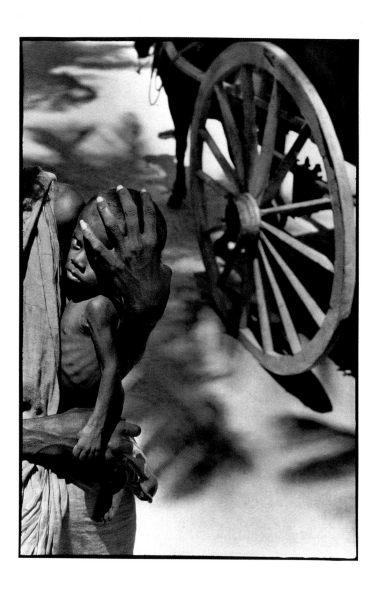

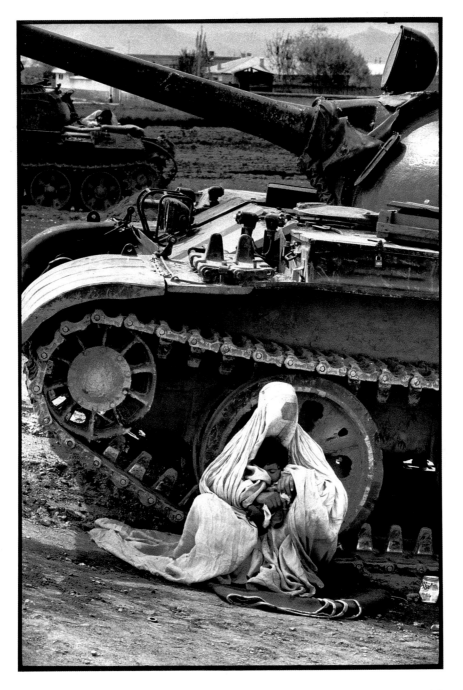

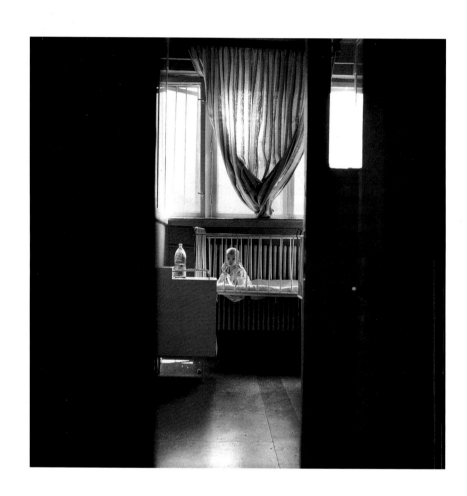

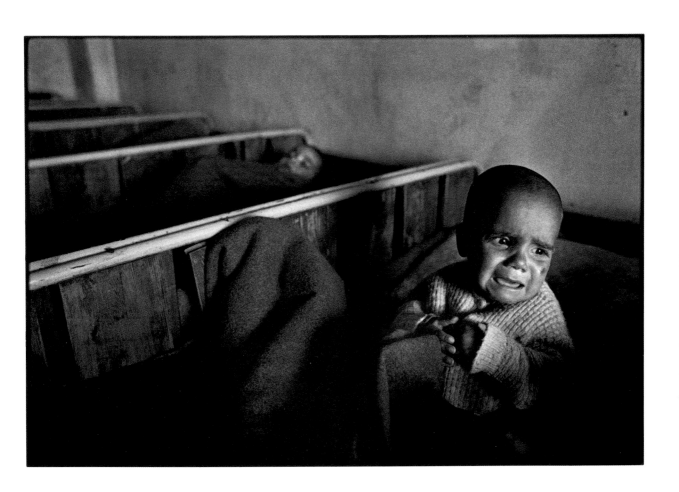

James Nachtwey, *Afghanistan,* 1996. | **53**

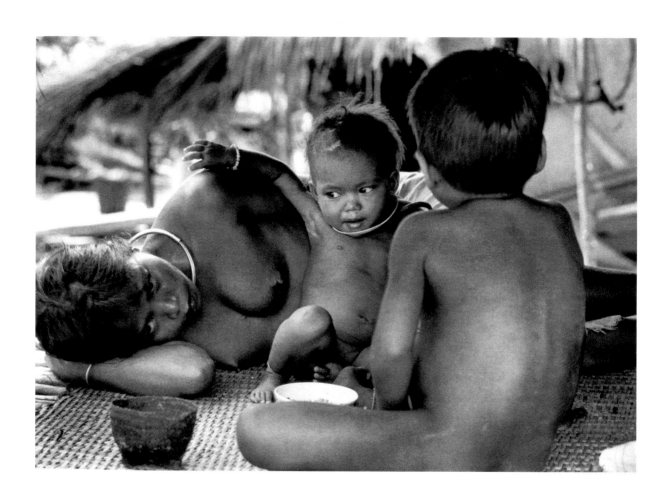

| Werner Bischof, Indo-China, *Indochine,* Indochina, 1952.

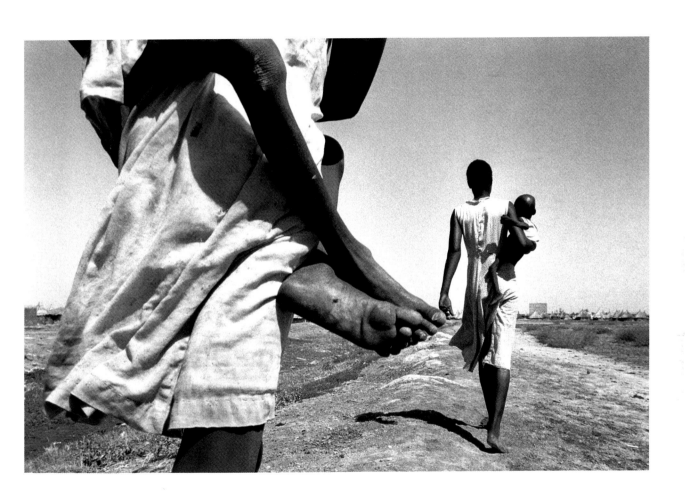

John Vink, Sudan, *Soudan,* 1988.

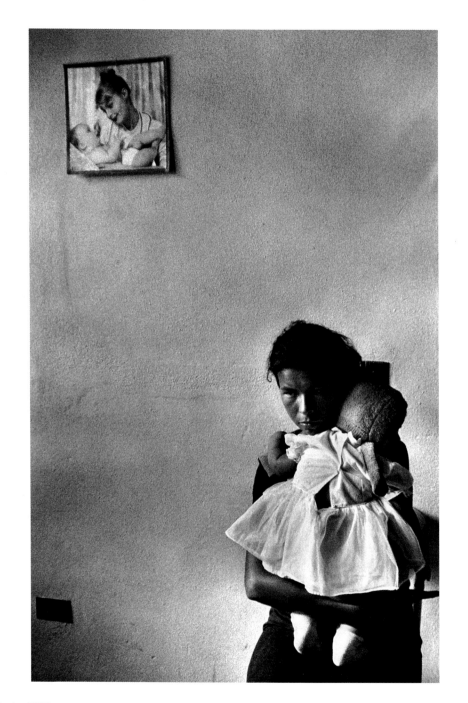

| Cornell Capa, *Salvador,* 1970.

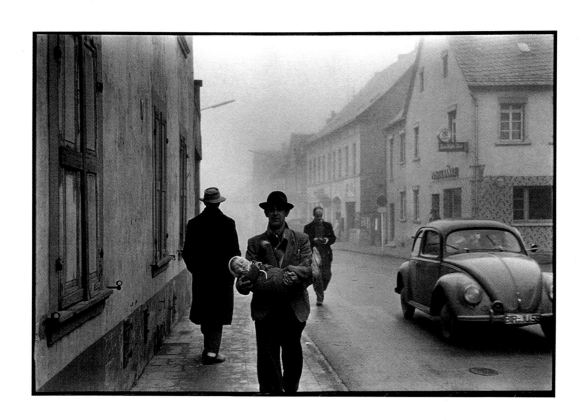

René Burri, Federal Republic of Germany, *RFA, Bundesrepublik Deutschland,* 1959. | **57**

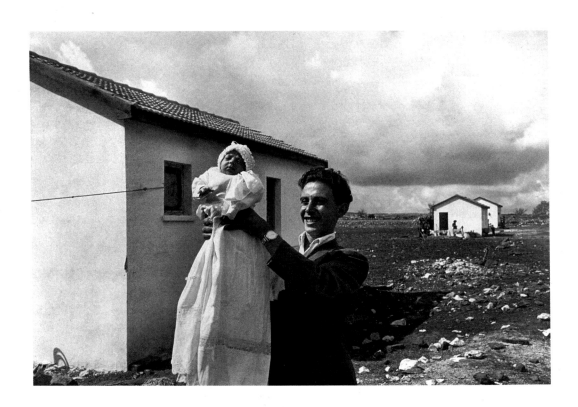

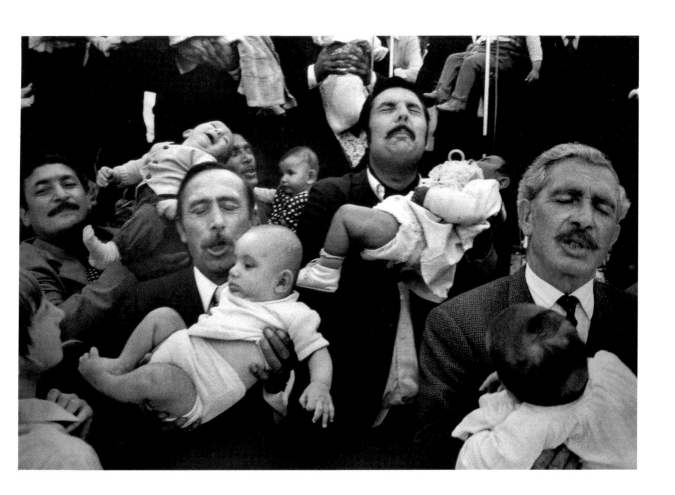

Josef Koudelka, *France,* Frankreich, 1970. **59**

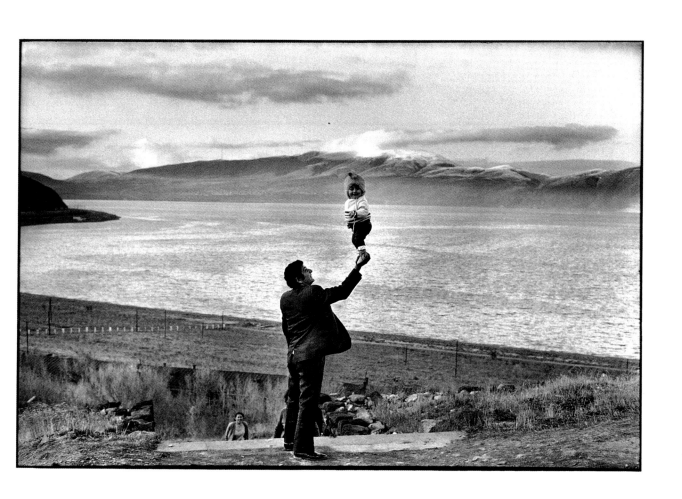

Henri Cartier-Bresson, USSR, *URSS,* UdSSR, 1972. |

Page 5 : *Paris, France.*
Josef Koudelka, 1986.
Seite 5: Paris, Frankreich.
Josef Koudelka, 1986.

Page 6-7: East 100th Street,
New York, USA.
Bruce Davidson, 1966-1968.
Page 6-7 : *100e rue Est,*
New York, États-Unis.
Bruce Davidson, 1966-1968.
Seite 6-7: East 100th Street,
New York, USA.
Bruce Davidson, 1966-1968.

Page 8 : *Ontario,*
Lambton County, Canada.
Larry Towell, 1989.
Seite 8: Ontario, Lambton
County, Kanada.
Larry Towell, 1989.

Page 9: Women of the Qusar
tribe watering tobacco plants.
Kordofan, Mesakin,
Southern Sudan.
George Rodger, 1949.
Page 9 : *Femmes de la tribu*
Qusar arrosant des plants
de tabac. Kordofan, Mesakin,
Sud-Soudan.
George Rodger, 1949.
Seite 9: Frauen des Stammes
Qusar, Tabakpflanzen
begießend. Kordofan,
Mesakin, Südsudan.
George Rodger, 1949.

Page 10: Prenatal visit.
South Africa.
Eve Arnold, 1973.
Page 10 : *Visite prénatale.*
Afrique du Sud.
Eve Arnold, 1973.
Seite 10: Mütterberatung.
Südafrika.
Eve Arnold, 1973.

Page 11 : *Paris, France.*
Patrick Zachmann, 1986.
Seite 11: Paris, Frankreich.
Patrick Zachmann, 1986.

Page 13: The pangs of
childbirth. USA.
Elliott Erwitt, 1972.
Page 13 : *Les douleurs avant*

l'accouchement. États-Unis.
Elliott Erwitt, 1972.
Seite 13: Wehen. USA.
Elliott Erwitt, 1972.

Page 14: Maternity hospital,
Caesarean section. Salvador.
Larry Towell, 1991.
Page 14 : *Maternité,*
département des césariennes.
Salvador.
Larry Towell, 1991.
Seite 14: Entbindungsstation,
Kaiserschnitt-Abteilung.
Salvador.
Larry Towell, 1991.

Page 15: Chicago,
Illinois, USA.
Wayne Miller, 1946.
Page 15 : *Chicago,*
Illinois, États-Unis.
Wayne Miller, 1946.
Seite 15: Chicago,
Illinois, USA.
Wayne Miller, 1946.

Page 17: *Paris, France.*
Josef Koudelka, 1986.
Seite 17: Paris, Frankreich.
Josef Koudelka, 1986.

Page 18: Israel.
Leonard Freed, 1973.
Page 18 : *Israël.*
Leonard Freed, 1973.
Seite 18: Israel.
Leonard Freed, 1973.

Page 19: Weighing time.
Xian, China.
Donovan Wylie, 1993.
Page 19 : *La pesée.*
Xian, Chine.
Donovan Wylie, 1993.
Seite 19: Wiegen.
Xian, China.
Donovan Wylie, 1993.

Page 20: New York, USA.
Elliott Erwitt, 1977.
Page 20 : *New York, États-Unis.*
Elliott Erwitt, 1977.
Seite 20: New York, USA.
Elliott Erwitt, 1977.

Page 21: Maternity ward
in the hospital at Montaigu.

Vendée, France.
Guy Le Querrec, 1972.
Page 21 : *Maternité de l'hôpital*
de Montaigu. Vendée, France.
Guy Le Querrec, 1972.
Seite 21: Entbindungdstation
im Krankenhaus von Montaigu.
Vendée, Frankreich.
Guy Le Querrec, 1972.

Page 22-23: New Delhi, India.
Raghu Rai, 1976.
Page 22-23: *New Delhi, Inde.*
Raghu Rai, 1976.
Seite 22-23: New Delhi,
Indien. Raghu Rai, 1976.

Page 24: Maternity ward at
Battambang hospital. Cambodia.
Patrick Zachmann, 1991.
Page 24 : *Maternité à l'hôpital*
de Battambang. Cambodge.
Patrick Zachmann, 1991.
Seite 24: Entbindungsstation
des Krankenhauses von
Battambang. Kambodscha.
Patrick Zachmann, 1991.

Page 25: Cardiff, Wales.
Josef Koudelka, 1969.
Page 25 : *Cardiff,*
Pays de Galles.
Josef Koudelka, 1969.
Seite 25: Cardiff, Wales.
Josef Koudelka, 1969.

Page 27: New York, USA.
Elliott Erwitt, 1953.
Page 27 : *New York, États-Unis.*
Elliott Erwitt, 1953.
Seite 27: New York, USA.
Elliott Erwitt, 1953.

Page 28: South Carolina, USA.
W. Eugene Smith, 1951.
Page 28 : *Caroline du Sud,*
États-Unis.
W. Eugene Smith, 1951.
Seite 28: South Carolina, USA.
W. Eugene Smith, 1951.

Page 29: Antalya, Turkey.
Marc Riboud, 1955.
Page 29 : *Antalya, Turquie.*
Marc Riboud, 1955.
Seite 29: Antalya, Türkei.
Marc Riboud, 1955.

Page 30: São Paulo,
Santos, Brazil.
Alex Majoli, 1996.
Page 30 : *São Paulo,*
Santos, Brésil.
Alex Majoli, 1996.
Seite 30: São Paulo,
Santos, Brasilien.
Alex Majoli, 1996.

Page 31: Alabama, USA.
Bruce Davidson, 1965.
Page 31 : *Alabama, États-Unis.*
Bruce Davidson, 1965.
Seite 31: Alabama, USA.
Bruce Davidson, 1965.

Page 32: *Niger.*
Raymond Depardon, 1989.
Seite 32: Niger.
Raymond Depardon, 1989.

Page 33: Calcutta, Bengal,
India. Marc Riboud, 1971.
Page 33 : *Calcutta, Bengale,*
Inde. Marc Riboud, 1971.
Seite 33: Kalkutta, Bengalen,
Indien. Marc Riboud, 1971.

Page 35: Mexico.
Henri Cartier-Bresson, 1934.
Page 35 : *Mexique.*
Henri Cartier-Bresson, 1934.
Seite 35: Mexiko.
Henri Cartier-Bresson, 1934.

Page 36: The Ruhr region,
Federal Republic of Germany.
René Burri, 1960.
Page 36 : *Région de la Ruhr,*
RFA. René Burri, 1960.
Seite 36: Ruhrgebiet,
Bundesrepublik Deutschland.
René Buri, 1960.

Page 37 : *Bougival,*
Yvelines, France.
Henri Cartier-Bresson, 1955.
Seite 37: Bougival,
Yvelines, Frankreich.
Henri Cartier-Bresson, 1955.

Page 38: Silver Lake, USA.
W. Eugene Smith, 1958.
Page 38 : *Silver Lake, États-*
Unis. W. Eugene Smith, 1958.
Seite 38: Silver Lake, USA.
W. Eugene Smith, 1958.

Page 39: Wales.
Bruce Davidson, 1965.
Page 39 : *Pays de Galles.*
Bruce Davidson, 1965.
Seite 39: Wales.
Bruce Davidson, 1965.

Page 40: USA.
Wayne Miller, 1948.
Page 40 : *États-Unis.*
Wayne Miller, 1948.
Seite 40: USA.
Wayne Miller, 1948.

Page 41: Pribaltiskaya Hotel.
Leningrad, Russia, USSR.
Carl De Keyzer, 1988.
Page 41 : *Hôtel Pribaltiskaya.*
Léningrad, Russie, URSS.
Carl De Keyzer, 1988.
Seite 41: Hotel Pribaltiskaya.
Leningrad, UdSSR.
Carl De Keyzer, 1988.

Page 42-43: Scotland.
Bruce Davidson, 1960.
Page 42-43 : *Écosse.*
Bruce Davidson, 1960.
Seite 42-43: Schottland.
Bruce Davidson, 1960.

Page 44-45: *Ontario,*
Lambton County, Canada.
Larry Towell, 1994.
Seite 44-45: Ontario, Lambton
County, Kanada.
Larry Towell, 1994.

Page 47: Extremadura, Spain.
David Seymour, 1936.
Page 47 : *Extremadure,*
Espagne.
David Seymour, 1936.
Seite 47: Estremadura,
Spanien.
David Seymour, 1936.

Page 48: Some of the thousand
orphans from the massacre,
guarded by soldiers of the
Rwandan Patriotic Army. Rwanda.
Paul Lowe, 1995.
Page 48 : *Quelques-uns*
des mille orphelins du massacre
sous la surveillance de soldats
de l'Armée patriotique
rwandaise. Rwanda.

Paul Lowe, 1995.
Seite 48: Einige der Tausend
Waisen nach dem Massaker
unter Aufsicht der Soldaten
der patriotischen Armee
Rwandas. Rwanda.
Paul Lowe, 1995.

Page 49: War in the Pacific;
a Marine with a wounded,
dying baby found in the moun-
tains of Saipan during the attack
on the island.
W. Eugene Smith, 1944.
Page 49 : *Guerre du Pacifique ;*
un marine avec un bébé blessé
et mourant trouvé dans les
montagnes de Saipan lors
de l'attaque sur l'île.
W. Eugene Smith, 1944.
Seite 49: Krieg im Pazifik;
ein Marine mit einem verletzen
sterbenden, in den
Saipan-Bergen bei dem Angriff
auf die Insel gefundenen
Babys.
W. Eugene Smith, 1944.

Page 50: Madurai,
Tamil nadu, India.
Henri Cartier-Bresson, 1949.
Page 50 : *Madurai,*
Tamil nadu, Inde.
Henri Cartier-Bresson, 1949.
Seite 50: Madurai,
Tamil nadu, Indien.
Henri Cartier-Bresson, 1949.

Page 51: Woman in a burgah.
Kabul, Afghanistan.
Abbas, 1992.
Page 51 : *Femme couverte*
du burgah. Kaboul, Afghanistan.
Abbas, 1992.
Seite 51: Burgah-verschleierte
Frau. Kabul, Afghanistan.
Abbas, 1992.

Page 52: Orphanage at
Constantza. Romania.
Raymond Depardon, 1990.
Page 52 : *Orphelinat de*
Constantza. Roumanie.
Raymond Depardon, 1990.
Seite 52: Waisenhaus von
Konstanza. Rumänien.

Raymon Depardon, 1990.

Page 53: Dormitory in the
central orphanage of Kabul.
Afghanistan.
James Nachtwey, 1996.
Page 53 : *Dortoir de l'orphelinat*
central de Kaboul. Afghanistan.
James Nachtwey, 1996.
Seite 53: Schlafsaal des
zentralen Waisenhauses,
Kabul. Afghanistan.
James Nachtwey, 1996.

Page 54: Hmong family.
Barau, Indochina.
Werner Bischof, 1952.
Page 54 : *Famille de Hmongs.*
Barau, Indochine.
Werner Bischof, 1952.
Seite 54: Eine Hmong-Familie.
Barau, Indochina.
Werner Bischof, 1952.

Page 55: Refugees from
southern Sudan.
Most of the children, suffering
from malnutrition, are too weak
to cover the three hundred yards
separating them from the
nutrition centre and have to be
carried there by their brothers
and sisters.
Kösti, Sudan. John Vink, 1988.
Page 55 : *Réfugiés du Sud-*
Soudan.
La plupart des enfants, souffrant
de malnutrition, sont trop faibles
pour parcourir les trois cents
mètres qui les séparent du
centre de nutrition et doivent
y être portés par leurs frères
et sœurs. Kösti, Soudan.
John Vink, 1988.
Seite 55: Flüchtlinge aus
dem Südsudan. Die meisten
unter Unternährung leidenden
Kinder sind zu schwach, um die
dreihundert Meter zur
Essensausgabe zu gehen und
müssen von ihren Brüdern und
Schwestern dorthin getragen
werden. Kösti, Sudan.
John Vink, 1988.

Page 56 : *Salvador.*

Cornell Capa, 1970.
Seite 56: Salvador.
Cornell Capa, 1970.

Page 57: Rhineland-Palatinate,
Federal Republic of Germany.
René Burri, 1959.
Page 57 : *Rhénanie, Palatinat,*
RFA.
René Burri, 1959.
Seite 57: Rheinland-Pfalz,
Bundesrepublik Deutschland.
René Burri, 1959.

Page 58: Newborn baby
in a camp of Jewish immigrants
from Italy. Israel.
David Seymour, 1951.
Page 58 : *Nouveau-né dans un*
camp d'immigrants juifs venus
d'Italie. Israël.
David Seymour, 1951.
Seite 58: Neugeborer in
einem Lager jüdischer
Einwanderer aus Italien. Israel.
David Seymour, 1951.

Page 59: Gypsies. Tours,
France.
Josef Koudelka, 1970.
Page 59 : *Gitans. Tours, France.*
Josef Koudelka, 1970.
Seite 59: Zigeuner.
Tours, Frankreich.
Josef Koudelka, 1970.

Page 61: Yerevan,
Armenia, USSR.
Henri Cartier-Bresson, 1972.
Page 61 : *Erevan, Arménie,*
URSS.
Henri Cartier-Bresson, 1972.
Seite 61: Eriwan, Armenien,
UdSSR.
Henri Cartier-Bresson,1972.